New Mother Quick Guide

2021 Baby Guide

Riley McMillan

Description

This book consists of twenty-five key tools to help new moms and moms-to-be with an extensive guide through pregnancy and motherhood during the pandemic.

Table of Contents

Introduction

Being a new mother during a pandemic will throw obstacles in your path every day which, normally, parents usually wouldn't even need to consider. For starters, there is a whole new vaccine that other pregnant people have never had to consider.

Having a pandemic baby has generally meant that parents have more time to spend with their newborn and less time and involvement from intrusive family and friends who don't always get the hint to give your new little family some space. A safe haven and a peace of mind, is a more viable excuse, to shy away from the scary reality us new moms face.

While you might not be able to have friends or family in your home, that doesn't have to mean you can't see them at all. In-person baby groups aren't on, but there are loads of online groups available and some of the relationships you build on there will prepare you for meeting up when the pandemic is over.

Despite all the changes that are happening in the world around you, now is not the time to panic. Instead, read on to learn these quick twenty-five key tips, tools, and reminders you need in order to navigate this uncertain world while handling the already life-altering situation of having a newborn. This body of work is a compilation of months of research, providing the latest and knowledgeable to date.

Chapter 1

Coronavirus Vaccine During Pregnancy

1. Understanding Why There Is A Lack of Trial Data

While there is plenty of data going around about any potential side effects that the vaccine may cause in the average adult, there is far less information about the vaccine and pregnant women. This is because it is not considered ethically correct to run trials on pregnant women and, as such, no data can be established in a quick and official manner.

Despite the lack of initial information regarding the vaccine concerning pregnancy, what data has since come to light shows that the benefits outweigh the negatives.

Many pregnant people (usually with their doctors' consent) are now choosing to have the vaccine but, as always, it is **entirely**

optional. Good news is that to date, women who participated in the vaccination process pre/post natal have not had any harm with becoming pregnant or keeping the pregnancy.

2. Antibodies For You and Your Baby

The good option to vaccinate, heavily outweigh the bad. We are seeing women who chose to have the vaccine during pregnancy record to the **CDC** that babies are born with **antibodies** for COVID-19 which are present in the placenta cord and breast milk. It is not yet known just how effective these antibodies are for the babies, as they are appearing in relatively small concentrations.

But it is still a good sign that they have gotten some protection from the virus once they have entered into the world. Additionally, the data coming in so far seems to imply that there is no increased risk of miscarriage, birth defects, and so on, than there would be without the presence of the vaccine.

3. Pregnant Women in High-Risk Categories

A valid reason you may choose to take the COVID-19 vaccine is because you are at a higher risk than the average pregnant woman.

In most areas, it has not yet been the case that pregnant women are deemed high risk based solely on the fact that they are with child.

Instead, women are more likely to be referred by their doctor and ultimately choose to get the vaccine if they are considered high risk for an alternative reason. The main two categories that apply here are either someone with an **underlying health condition or someone who works in a public-facing role** that cannot be prevented. Keep in mind pregnant women with **COVID-19** had adverse pregnancy outcomes such as **preterm birth**. It is a classic case of how the safety of the mother outweighs the potential risk to the unborn baby. Fortunately, as we have seen, the risk to the baby seems very little when vaccinated, so it is definitely better to be safe than sorry!

4. V-Safe Program

Ultimately, if you do decide to have the vaccine, then there is a way you can help other expectant mothers feel safe to do so in the future, too. The CDC has a system called the V- **safe program**, which they have adapted to include an additional subcategory: the v-safe COVID-19 **vaccine pregnancy registry**.

As with the v-safe program as a whole, the pregnancy registry is completely voluntary and you can opt out anytime.Any woman that enrolls in the v-safe program and was pregnant at the time of being vaccinated or within thirty days after can sign up for the pregnancy option.

If you are in the program, you will be regularly contacted throughout your pregnancy and potentially an additional time, roughly three months after your baby's birth.

The main things the CDC is trying to check are: whether you develop any pregnancy conditions such as preeclampsia or gestational diabetes, if you have any issues during the birth, and finally, if there are any issues with your newborn — for example, preterm labor or low birth weight. This information is vital to helping the CDC, doctors, and other pregnant women in continuing to make an informed decision about the vaccine going forward.

Chapter 2:

Vitamins and Medicines

5. Prenatal Vitamins For Every Pregnant Mom

Prenatal vitamins help fill any gaps in your diet where you might not be getting enough of the right stuff to provide the best environment for your baby. It is much easier to get too few of a vitamin than it is to get too much.

Therefore, choosing to supplement your diet has very little chance of doing you any harm, even if it turns out you already get enough of each vitamin via your food intake. At a minimum, it is suggested that you take six hundred units of **vitamin D** and four hundred milligrams of **folic acid** a day since these are the core vitamins needed for healthy growth and development. Beyond these two, the other highly suggested supplements include **calcium, iron, and Omega-3**. Generally speaking to make it simpler on yourself and ensure you are getting an adequate dose of all the correct ones, choose to buy brands specifically designed for pregnant women.

Pandemic based thoughts and eating habits also need to be considered as eating more oranges and grapefruit will help you load up on the much needed vitamin c power. Healthy bright vegetables, whole grains, dairy, and eating small meals through out the day can help fight boredom, anxiety, and cravings during lock down.

6. Other Prenatal Medication You Might Encounter

Whether there is a specific medical condition occurring during your pregnancy or a family history of risks, you might find that you have to take additional medication besides the standard prenatal vitamins while you are pregnant.

For a few of the common conditions, such as preeclampsia and hypertension, a **low dose of aspirin** is prescribed to be taken on a daily basis as a preventative measure. Make sure you discuss this with your Healthcare provider first to ensure optimum care. High-risk pregnancies are mostly recognized by either being of an older maternal age, or your mother or sister(s) have a history of these risks. Should you develop nearly any pregnancy-related conditions, you will be put on an appropriate medication that will then be re-evaluated after you have given birth. For example, gestational diabetes results in tablets or insulin shots, while anti hypertensive medication is given for gestational hypertension and preeclampsia.

Be sure to talk with your healthcare provider if you develop any of these conditions, they will know best the appropriate options.

Remember to eat immune boosting foods that are safe for baby that ensure proper nutrient intake, natural fruit and protein and salad greens, eggs and dairy. Covid-19 gives us a rare opportunity to pay closer attention to these types of food, and not just giving into cravings or over indulging. Instead women are forced to pay closer attention to those vitamin c and iron enriched foods, that allows proper defense and nutrients for baby and from the virus. Now is the time to get creative in the kitchen and naturally healthy.

7. Continuing to Take Prenatal Vitamins Postnatally

Taking prenatal vitamins after you have given birth is less of a requirement compared with your actual pregnancy. However, there are a lot of **benefits** in continuing to do so. For starters, your body will have just lost a significant amount of tissue, cells, and blood.

In fact, for weeks to months after birth, you will still be losing blood. Prenatal vitamins contain all the right to help your body restore what it has lost and is continuing to lose, ideally even helping to speed up your recovery.

Similarly, your immune system is going to be a bit out of shape due to the nature of your body growing a completely different human for the last nine months. Again, the supplements in your prenatal vitamins will help your immune system settle back down to normal in no time.

Natural pre/postnatal vitamins to consider are **Ritual** and **EU Natural** they have a all natural, vegan feel with non fillers, which are safe for mom and baby.Prenatal vitamins can be extra helpful if you are breastfeeding just like during pregnancy, taking prenatal vitamins while breastfeeding will increase lactation, therefore help supply your baby with the vitamins they need for healthy growth.

Remember it is important to get enough Vitamin D to aid in self isolation depression and lack of sunlight post pregnancy.

The vitamin also helps immune cells produce antibodies, which aid in the prevention of infections. This of course is particularly relevant during COVID-19 and pregnancy.

8. Other Medication You Might Require Postnatally

Sometimes doctors recommend that you start on additional **iron supplements** postpartum to prevent you from becoming anemic while your body readjusts. In these cases, you will want to have **stool softeners** at the ready or be prepared to pump your diet full of fiber, as iron has a nasty side effect: it makes you incredibly constipated.

There are also scenarios where you may need additional medication postpartum, regardless of whether you required anything extra during your pregnancy. For starters, if you experienced high blood pressure, you will still be on your medication for at least two weeks post-birth. Preeclampsia is another one you would need continued monitoring for; in fact, it can even appear postnatally despite having no signs of it prior. Another major issue some women need medication for is **clotting**. Every woman will have some clotting after they have given birth; it is a core part of how the body functions in removing so much excess tissue, blood, and so on.

However, some mothers are at risk of a more dangerous form of clotting. Those in the high-risk category include women who have a history or family history of these sorts of clots, women over 35 years of age, overweight women, and women who have given birth to multiples. There are additional factors besides these but these are the most common. There are numerous ways to reduce the risk but it will be via daily injections if your doctor chooses to deal with it preemptively.

Depending on the risk, these can either be **anticoagulant** based to prevent the clots from fully forming or an alternative medication that causes the uterus to contract quicker than it would have by itself. The latter helps prevent clots by returning your uterus to its original size sooner, at which point the chance of clots is dramatically reduced. Speak with your Healthcare provider regarding **pre/post natal** issues and your **vaccination**, being safer than worried is indeed what us women strive for!

9. Vitamins For Your Baby

Upon their birth, with your permission, your baby will receive a vitamin K shot. This shot is to prevent the occurrence of **vitamin K deficient bleeding (VKDB)**, a condition that can appear anytime in the first six months of your baby's life if no preventative measures are taken.

Vitamin K is primarily found in our food, which is why it is harder for babies to always get enough. Beyond their birth, it is also highly   recommended that you supplement your baby with other vitamins.

Ideally, both **breastmilk and formula** will contain all the necessary vitamins, but this is not always the case, so it is safer to supplement from   the get-go.Fortunately, there is a big market for multivitamins for babies and toddlers.

At such a young age, they will need to be taking the supplements in liquid form. If you are not sure which brand or product to choose, then the main thing is to check that it offers ample amounts of **(400IU) vitamin D**, as this continues to be the most important vitamin for your baby's development.

Other vitamins you want to look for are vitamin C, vitamin A, iron, Omega-3, and fluoride (this one is in preparation for when their teeth start showing up). Ensure at all times, check with your Healthcare provider, for the the most optimum care.

Chapter 3:

How to Social Distance
With A Baby

10. Virtual Celebrations and Events

Although the pandemic has put many of our social plans on hold, it doesn't mean you can't still have virtual celebrations of your upcoming bundle of joy. Pregnant women are considered to be at a higher risk than average during the Coronavirus pandemic, so staying home is the safest option for you and your baby. Luckily, there are plenty of games and other activities that can be played via a video call, still making the events enjoyable for all who join.

Most games that go down well during virtual baby showers and gender reveals rely heavily on being visually engaging. Some of the best games consist of **"Who's That Baby?"** and **"Guess the Number,"** while other activities, such as " **Baby**

Bingo" and " **Baby Shower Jeopardy**" as well as the guest book, are easily adapted to an online format. Depending on your local restrictions and the ability of your family and friends to get tested, there is also the option that you could hold an outdoor function for your celebrations.However, even with masks, social distancing, and an outdoor space, nothing will prevent you from contracting the virus as much as not attending events with people present.

11. Visitors and Your Newborn

Generally speaking, you have two main options in terms of visitors during a pandemic. The first is that everyone who is planning on coming into your house has to quarantine for the two weeks prior in order to significantly reduce the risk of having been exposed themselves. The other is that no one enters your premises until after the pandemic is over. The second option does not mean people can't meet or see your baby, but it does mean that there won't be any holding or physical help involved. The easiest way to navigate the fact that people can't enter your home is to meet up with them somewhere outside, including a garden, if your visitors can access it without passing through the house.

Otherwise, have "drive-by" visits, where your visitors can say hello from outside your window while your baby is safely on the other side. If all else fails, we are lucky enough to live in a time where technology makes it remarkably easy to keep in contact. Therefore, it may be more straightforward to video call those that matter most to make that all-important first introduction. If nothing else, it is particularly easy to send out photos and videos to all those you want to keep in the loop.

12. Online Baby Groups

Groups are just as crucial for moms and dads as they are for your baby. Being able to catch up with other parents who are experiencing the same things around the same time as you are is essential to maintaining your sanity during the early stages of your child's life.

Unfortunately, the coronavirus has put this sort of socializing largely on hold.

However, there are a few methods in place to combat this issue. In some areas, there is the availability of virtual baby groups or, at minimum, groups involving video calls so that the babies all get the opportunity to smile and laugh with others roughly their age.

Worth mentioning are **gymboree play online classes**, or **Happity** who will match you with providers in your area. Fortunately, online platforms for parents have been around since long before the pandemic began. Therefore, it is remarkably easy to find one and join a group that is local to you or centered around your interests.

Online groups are also the perfect way to get to know each other and reduce some of the awkwardness when you finally get around to meeting up in person.

13. Childcare

There is no correct answer for what you should choose to do when it comes to childcare during a pandemic. On the one hand, family or friends might seem like the obvious choice. The upside to relatives is that you could consider quarantining together and there is a reduced risk of exposure to the virus since there will be significantly fewer other children than at a daycare or similar group. The downside of relying on family is that you risk the virus spreading to them due to you being back out in the workforce.

Another point to consider family and friends do not have the same legal and financial responsibilities as registered childcare places, meaning that they may not follow coronavirus guidelines as strictly or not always be available when you need them to be. Evidently, your other option is a daycare or a similar type of setting.

The issue with a nursery is that your child will be coming into contact with a lot of other people, both adults and children. This naturally increases the risk of them being exposed to,and bringing home, the virus. However, day-cares and the like have CDC-approved protocols that they are required to put in place for the duration of the pandemic. Generally, this covers things such as screening all those arriving for any signs and symptoms, having staff wear masks at all times, and increased sanitization and cleaning efforts, to name but a few.

Chapter 4:

Hygiene Practices

14. General Hygiene and Hand Washing

Keeping yourself clean is the surest way to maintain your baby's overall hygiene too. Baby's only need a bath once to twice a week, so by remaining clean, you are making sure that your child isn't being exposed to any unnecessary germs or bacteria in the meantime. Not only that but in keeping yourself washed you will find that you have a clearer mind and feel more energized to deal with the unrelenting torrent of care that your baby requires of you. Additionally, regular **hand washing** is a must anytime but is even more crucial during a pandemic.

Having anyone who plans on being around your baby wash their hands before each interaction is a good idea. It's also not a bad idea to wash your baby's hands now and then—they are constantly putting them in their mouths and sometimes we don't consider all the places those little hands could have touched or been touched. While we are in a pandemic, you might be tempted to use sanitizer on your baby's hands just as you do your own while out and about. However, this is highly inadvisable. Baby skin is extremely sensitive and cannot handle the chemicals and similar products that even the most sensitive sanitizers consist of.

Fortunately, having a baby around means you will always have **baby wipes** on hand, perfect for keeping their hands clean.

15. Keeping Baby Clean Day And Night

When it comes to keeping your baby clean, everyone is aware of the pain of a parent's existence, which is changing diapers. Diaper changes should be taking place roughly every two hours unless you notice that it is already full and dirty before then. Regularly changing your baby's diaper goes beyond basic cleanliness.

As their skin is so delicate, it takes no time at all for them to begin to get a rash from prolonged dampness or contact with solids. Diaper creams go a long way to holding off the worst but once a rash starts, it can get bad very quickly. So, it is much safer to be preventative by changing your baby's diaper often.

You also want to make sure you are washing your baby's clothes often enough. They might seem clean if you haven't had to deal with your child spitting up, vomiting, or managing to explode out of their diaper. In reality, with how fragile babies' immune systems are, if your child has worn it for more than a day or two, it is best to put it through a wash.

Finally, regardless of how often you change your own bedding, you are going to want to change your baby's every day or two, aside from an reaction to spills, diaper blowouts, and similar. As with their clothing, this is primarily a result of babies being delicate. As a result, problems can arise from them spending too much time in an area covered in germs.

Their bedding may not seem particularly dirty but babies are messy! They will often dribble in their sleep and this alone is enough to introduce a lot of potentially harmful bacteria to their sleeping area.

16. Breast Cleanliness

Keeping your breasts and nipples clean is relevant for all expectant mothers. Even if you have no intentions of breastfeeding, your body will still produce milk at some point.

You should plan to keep the area adequately cleaned to reduce the chances of any infections and prevent the area from additional itchiness.

In fact, for many mothers, breast milk starts to make an appearance before the birth of their baby. The best way to deal with milky breasts is to wash them gently with warm, clean water.

Choose not to wash them with soap, as this can add to the chances of you experiencing irritation or infections. Aside from cleaning, your nipples they will also respond well to being aired out. They are not used to feeling damp constantly, so airing them out helps them feel refreshed and similarly reduces the likelihood of irritation.

While it is vital that you keep your breasts in good condition, there is a straightforward way to ensure that your milk has as little impact on your clothes as possible: breast pads. They aren't going to stop milk from getting all over your nipples, but they are a lifesaver both day and night in terms of keeping your clothes from getting soaked.

You can opt for either disposable or reusable types of breast pads. Both types are easy and practical to use! Even so, it is best to aim to change your nursing bra every day or two if you are breastfeeding. This is primarily because milk can get everywhere while your baby feeds, often without you even noticing. Since this can lead to smelly bras, if nothing worse, it is well worth investing in at least two nursing bras, so it is easy to swap them out regularly.

In a similar vein, make sure to always wash your breast pump after each use. This might sound a little time-consuming, but it is much more worthwhile to spend time cleaning it than risk your baby being exposed to dangerous bacteria.

On another note if your looking for lactation support, the online community has **Lactation Support Groups**, Telehealth or app's such as **Maple(get maple.ca).** These online programs offer a live **Lactation Consultant** in your area who would be able to either come to your home or provide virtual appointments.

17. Steering Clear of Scented Washing Products

Not only are scented washing products a bad call for your newborn but you should generally avoid them during pregnancy .

While pregnant, your private regions are much more sensitive to changes in your vaginal pH level than usual. In both cases, it is best to avoid unnecessarily chemical-heavy products.

For your private regions, it is advised that you stick to only washing with water, while you should ideally wash your baby with a sensitive soap designed for the delicate pH balance of their skin.For pregnant women, throwing off your pH balance can cause all sorts of ailments including vaginal thrush, while for your baby it can aggravate conditions such as eczema.

Chapter 5:

Mommy and Baby Survival Tips

18. Take It One Day At A Time

Being a parent is an experience that you get very little hands-on preparation for. To throw a pandemic on top of that is only going to create even higher levels of stress and anxiety within household. Therefore, it is essential to regularly remind yourself of how good a job you are doing. To make it through each day with a newborn is one incredible feat; no one has an easy time with newborns and if they claim otherwise, then chances are their newborn is not a newborn anymore and they have repressed the worst of it. When you find yourself struggling, the best thing you can do is reward yourself with words of encouragement.

Let yourself know what a good job you have done getting through each particular day. Do this every day and, before you know it, time will have flown by. You also don't have to be the only one telling you what a good job you are doing; family, friends, and online parent groups are all great places to receive positive comments, too.

19. Prioritizing Baby

When you have your baby, you will probably experience what most people refer to as 'baby brain.' For many, this phenomenon can last anywhere up to a year. Simply put, it is the result of all your energy and hormones being laser-focused on your baby's needs, causing your brain to stop functioning entirely like normal. It is nothing concerning, just little things like finding it harder to pay attention to conversations going on around you—or even involving you—or forgetting the word for something simple like "table."

Given that all your focus and attention is on your new child, as it should be, you should realize that the idea of entertaining guests and

other people's agendas simply because they want to meet the baby is not your responsibility at this time. With a newborn, the priority of those around you should be to see when you are free to introduce your baby and not trying to force you to fit into their timetable instead.

On the plus side, with the pandemic, if you absolutely don't want to see anyone and want to focus solely on your baby for a while, you have the perfect excuse to keep people at bay.

Study show there is no need for stimulating actions for the first couple of months, so no need to feel guilty that baby is not getting enough stimulation. However be sure that as baby grows **tummy time,** singing and talking to baby is ideal for early development and attachment.

20. Bonding Time

Bonding is so important in your child's life and it starts from the moment they are born.

Being a mom likely means that, in those first weeks to months of your child's life, you are the primary caregiver and, as such, the one who the baby will naturally begin to bond with more swiftly. There is nothing negative about this. It is the intended purpose of your time with your child but there are two things to be aware of.

The first is that it is entirely normal if you do not immediately feel a burst of love and attachment towards your baby. This is often overplayed and can make mothers feel bad when it doesn't occur.

But think about it logically, this is a whole new person that you only just met, you can't expect it to be love at first sight—but don't worry, those feelings of love will soon come. However, if you especially feel like you're struggling, be sure to contact your doctor as you could be experiencing postpartum depression.

The second thing to be aware of is how much bonding time your partner is getting with your new baby.

Baby's need time to bond with both their parents, so make sure that your partner is getting some one-on-one time when they're home. The silver lining of the pandemic is that there is a high chance that you or your partner are working from, or generally at, home.

Therefore, both parents have a more immediate presence in your child's daily routine, helping to cement these bonds. Bonding between parents and their baby is of the utmost importance, but so is maintaining the bond between the parents.

Talking to your partner and making sure that the two of you remember to spend time together is just as crucial to a happy, functioning household as getting to grips with how to parent. However, don't put all the pressure of maintaining this relationship on yourself.

Your partner should be just as intent on bringing the focus back to the two of you from time to time. It may be pertinent to have a conversation before your baby arrives about how you plan to make sure you both remember to interact with each other.

Key tips would be to **create and maintain a structured routine, as well as be flexible. Strive to be kind, and apologize when you loose control, and remember to ask for help when needed.**

21. Remember to Eat

Your baby is relying on you to survive. Therefore, there are few things more important than making sure you eat. Just to be clear, the only things more important are making sure your baby is safe and that you are trying to get enough sleep. The point is, if you eat and keep yourself healthy, it is one hundred times easier to make sure that your baby is on track too.

With how exhausting babies are and how much of our focus they require, eating while being a parent is the most important part of your day. Eating is the only way to ensure you have both the **mental and physical energy** to get through the day and see to all your baby's needs.

This reality is only doubled if you are also breastfeeding or pumping. While lots of people may have joked about you eating for two while pregnant, it is now that the term really begins to apply. The food you consume is the basis for all the nutrients your child is getting, so even if you are supplementing with multivitamins, putting effort into eating enough is the best thing you can do for your baby.

Not only that, but breastfeeding will also drain you of your fluids, so keep yourself topped up with liquids to stave off any chances of **becoming dehydrated** while also increasing your chances of having high levels of supply.

22. Get Outside

Despite the reasonable concern that taking your baby anywhere during a pandemic will put them at risk, it is still essential that you and your baby get outside for some fresh air. Leaving your house doesn't have to result in going anywhere specific. It is easy to stop yourself and your baby from being exposed to the virus by keeping your outside activities to places such as the park and other locations where

it is incredibly simple to keep your distance from anyone else who is enjoying some time away from home.Getting out and about and soaking up some fresh air is the perfect way to handle feeling a multitude of negative emotions. Outdoor activities ensure that you get a nice full dose of vitamin D, even on a cloudy day. Additionally, it has been known for years now that fresh air does something fantastic to our health, both physically and mentally—so who wouldn't want to get out in it with their newborn in tow. Heading outside is also a great way of calming a baby who is struggling to settle. It turns out that being outdoors is the perfect way to destress anyone, regardless of their age.

23. Don't Stress Over Housework

Being a parent can, at times, feel like you are barely managing to stay on top of things. This is a totally normal feeling to have, being one that is experienced by every parent at some early stage of their child's life. For this reason, you have to make sure you do not start stressing out over housework. Some chores are necessary but, when you come to prioritizing, you will learn that plenty are not as important as you were once led to believe. The really essential things to make sure you do include are keeping yourself and your baby fed, clean, and clothed.

Anything beyond that is a plus. If you find that you don't have time to wash up every day or you have not touched the laundry in three days, that's fine! One way to think about it is this: imagine all the things on your to-do list are juggling balls, some made of glass, others of plastic. The glass balls cannot be dropped—they consist of feeding, washing, getting enough sleep, and any other priority that is an actual essential in your household. The plastic balls are everything else. You can drop them from time to time and it won't have any lasting effect; you can just pick them up later.

24. Accept Help When You Need It

Remember you are not expected to be perfect, remind yourself, its all about mommy and baby health. Be aware of your own emotion at least once a day, if you become overwhelmed its perfectly ok to allow your partner to help.

Accepting help when you need it is key to maintaining your sanity during the first couple of months of living with a newborn.

While it may be difficult to picture how you can get any help from people outside your household during a pandemic, there are ways. Bear in mind, just because people can't necessarily come into your home, it doesn't mean that you can't receive some of the same help you would have otherwise. Expected Friends and family can still drop off cooked meals, go and get some shopping at the groceries or run an errand or two for you. The people around you would usually love to help out and, if it keeps you and your baby home and safe, all the better! **Reminder: Asymptomatic infections remain a priority** and as so, Maternal anxiety and stress have been shown to affect pre/postmartum so be sure to connect with a Mental Health therapist if needs be through your **OBGYN** or local hospital where delivered.

25. Schedule Some 'Me' Time

Ideally, your 'me' time will be singled out for you to enjoy by yourself but don't feel like you can't have some 'me' time with your baby tagging along. The key part of any 'me' time is to do something that you know you will enjoy. This is something you would do with some regularity before your child's birth but you haven't found the time to do it since. Having some time to yourself, doing something enjoyable, is paramount to maintaining a healthy mental state. This is even more essential during a pandemic. Due to the nature of being home more with less opportunity for visitors, there is a much higher chance that you will not experience natural break from being the center of your baby's world. Typically, this would occur when grandparents or others came to visit. Therefore, it is paramount in a time where our mental health is already at risk (global pandemic concerns plus the usual pregnancy and postpartum hormones), that you put in the effort to take a safe step back when you need to. Being in a pandemic doesn't have to mean you are alone. There are social media sites that cater to motherhood such as **Social.Mom(App)** as well as **The leaky boob, Pink and Blue, Black Moms Connection,** are just to name a few.

If you have a partner at home with you, take turns being the solo parent from time to time; if you live alone with your baby, perhaps ask someone to come over.

They can still take your little one out for a walk—it doesn't have to last more than twenty minutes and the chances of your baby being exposed to the virus won't be any higher than if you were to take them on the walk yourself. Also, once settled you may want to work on getting your **pregnant body** back, its about feeling good physical and mentally. Be sure to check yor local area for online fitness classes designed for postpartum moms and babies such as **Baby Bee Yoga,** and **The Mama Reset**.

Conclusion

With any luck, you will feel more prepared for all the changes that are headed your way after reading this. Hopefully, you are more aware of how to face the parenting challenge during a pandemic. Also armed with a bit of common knowledge information you can begin to notice that a pandemic doesn't have to result in a significant impact on your parenting as you might have first suspected. What is important is that we all pay attention to what changes the coronavirus has caused us to implement but not to let it detract from such an extraordinary time in your and your baby's life.

Be sure to check with your pediatrician on whether to bring the baby to wellness visits, or go virtual. A video visit may be more ideal given the climate, as the doctor can assess any issues visually and roadblocks with breastfeeding. Parenting was never going to be easy but, by learning the basics and getting the hang of them during such a tumultuous time, will likely mean that the future will feel like a walk in the park once the pandemic is all over. The main thing you need to remember is: do not panic. You will succeed with the support of those around you. So try to relax and spend this time enjoying your baby.

References

Achwal, A. (December 7, 2018). *Blood clots after delivery - symptoms and treatment.* FirstCry Parenting.

https://parenting.firstcry.com/articles/blood-clots-after-delivery-symptoms-and-treatment/

Aviva Romm. (n.d.). *Prenatal vitamins: do you need one and how to choose.* Aviva

Romm MD. https://avivaromm.com/prenatal-vitamins/

Centers for Disease Control and Prevention. (April 6, 2021). *V-safe COVID-19 vaccine pregnancy registry.*

www.cdc.gov/coronavirus/2019-ncov/vaccines/safety/vsafepregnancyregistry.html

Donor Egg Bank USA. (August 30, 2019). *Are you at risk? What you need to know about high-risk pregnancies.*

donoreggbankusa.com/resources/blog/know-about-high-risk-pregnancies

Enfamil. (n.d.). *Vitamins for babies: what vitamins do babies need?*

www.enfamil.com/articles/vitamins-for-babies/

Healthline. (n.d.). *Child care challenges: how are parents managing in the pandemic?*

www.healthline.com/health/parenting/child-care-challenges-how-are-parents-managing-due-to-the-pandemic

Hilton-Andersen, C., E. Bacharach, & J. Gomez. (September 30, 2020). *The thirteen best prenatal vitamins for soon-to-be moms, according to experts.* Women's Health.

www.womenshealthmag.com/health/a21288517/best-prenatal-vitamins/

Julee. (n.d.). *Five hygiene tips for new mothers.* Mommy's Memorandum.

https://mommysmemorandum.com/5-hygiene-tips-mothers/

Karten, M.M. (April, 2018). *Why do newborns need a vitamin K shot?* Kids Health.

https://kidshealth.org/en/parents/vitamin-k-shot.html

March of Dimes. (November 24, 2020). *Bringing your new baby home during the coronavirus pandemic.* News Moms Need.

https://newsmomsneed.marchofdimes.org/coronavirus/bringing-your-new-baby

-home-during-the-coronavirus-pandemic/

Marissa. (February 5, 2018). *Prenatal vitamins before, during, and after pregnancy.*

We Have Kids.

https://wehavekids.com/having-baby/Prenatal-Vitamins-Before-During-and-After-Pregnancy

Medical News Today. (February 26, 2018). *Postpartum blood clots and bleeding: what to expect.*
www.medicalnewstoday.com/articles/321046

Migala, J. (November 18, 2020). *How to have a virtual baby shower.* What To Expect.

www.whattoexpect.com/news/pregnancy/virtual-baby-showers/

Mother To Baby. (April 13, 2021). *COVID-19 vaccines.*

https://mothertobaby.org/fact-sheets/covid-19-vaccines/

National Institute for Health and Care Excellence (NICE). (June 25, 2019).

Hypertension in pregnancy: diagnosis and management.

www.nice.org.uk/guidance/ng133/chapter/Recommendations#management-of-gestational-hypertension

New Kids Center. (n.d.). *Six main types of vitamins for babies.* www.newkidscenter.org/Vitamins-For-Babies.html

Pansare, U. (November 15, 2018). *Hygiene tips all pregnant women and new moms must follow.* The Health Site. www.thehealthsite.com/parenting/baby-care/hygiene-tips-all-pregnant-women-and-new-moms-must-follow-623608/

Poirier, K. (November 14, 2019). *Baby's first year, eleven survival tips for a new mom.* Mama Sloth. https://mamasloth.com/babys-first-year-11-survival-tips-for-new-moms/

Sarma, J. (April 17, 2020). *Hygiene rules that every mom must follow for her baby in the times of COVID-19.* The Health Site. www.thehealthsite.com/parenting/baby-care/hygiene-rules-that-every-mom-must-follow-for-her-baby-in-the-times-of-covid-19-739956/

The First Time Mamma. (February 3, 2020). *Ten life-changing new mom survival tips.* https://thefirsttimemamma.com/new-mom-survival-tips/

US Department of Health and Human Services. (November 19, 2018). *What are the treatments for preeclampsia, eclampsia, & HELLP syndrome?* NICHD.

www.nichd.nih.gov/health/topics/preeclampsia/conditioninfo/treatments